LEAN AND GREEN
DIET

Table of Content

INTRODUCTION

Consumers have long been drawn to the convenience of meal replacement diets that take the guesswork out of weight loss. One popular meal replacement plan is the Optavia Diet. By combining "fuelings" (shakes, bars, and other pre-packaged foods) with a six-small-meals-per-day philosophy, the Optavia Diet aims to help people lose weight by consuming small amounts of calories throughout the day. Optavia adds a social support component by offering access to a health coach who can answer questions and provide encouragement.

To help you decide if the program could help you achieve your weight loss goals, here's a look at how the Optavia Diet works, as well as the plan's pros and cons. The Optavia diet is a meal replacement plan. Followers eat a certain number of 'fuelings' per day (plus one homemade meal) resulting in calorie reduction and weight loss. Experts worry that it's unsustainable; many will regain weight when transitioning off the meal replacements.

The Optavia Diet might sound unfamiliar, as the name itself hasn't been around very long. You're more likely to have heard of the diet by its previous name, Take Shape for Life, which was rebranded as Optavia in July 2017. Take Shape for Life began as a subsidiary of Medifast, a weight-loss product company founded in 1980 by a medical doctor named Dr. William Vitale. When it was introduced in 2002, the intent of Take Shape for Life was to offer Medifast's products in an online format better suited to the digital age. The Optavia Diet is not intended for a specific audience, but it tends to appeal to people who want to stop "overthinking" an eating plan.

With Optavia's popular "5 & 1" plan, five out of the six small meals per day are pre-planned and pre-packaged, eliminating the need for any big decisions when it's time to eat. Optavia tends to be a favorite among people with a busy lifestyle, but the plan's reduced-calorie approach is intended for anyone looking to lose weight. Still, the Optavia Diet has not been without controversy. Critics have called the plan a pyramid scheme because of its multi-level structure, and the sales and promotions aspect of the program can be a turnoff for potential customers.

How to Spot a Weight Loss Scam

Users who complete Optavia's program are encouraged to become coaches, sell the company's products, and recruit new sales representatives.

L ike other meal replacement diets, the Optavia Diet provides users with its own array of branded products that take the place of several meals throughout the day. Optavia offers diet plans for goals of weight loss and weight maintenance.

The "5 & 1" plan is the most popular and is designed for rapid weight loss. On this plan, users eat five of Optavia's "fuelings" and one low-calorie "lean and green" homemade meal per day. Optavia's other plans, the "3 & 3" and "4 & 2 & 1", combine "real" meals with meal replacements. These plans are best-suited to users who want to lose weight slowly or maintain their current weight.

On all of Optavia's plans, both "fuelings" and "lean and green" homemade meals are kept within strict calorie ranges.

T he Optavia Diet deviates from health and nutrition guidelines encouraged by the United States Department of Agriculture (USDA) in several areas.

The USDA's Dietary Guidelines for Americans 2015-2020 estimate that a healthy adult requires 1600 to 3000 calories per day, depending on their activity level. Although Optavia's 5 & 1 plan is intended for weight loss, the 800 to 1000 calorie count per day is an extreme reduction from the USDA's recommendation.

One area where Optavia deviates from USDA recommendations is in terms of macronutrients specifically, carbohydrates. Optavia's plans reportedly provide 80 to 100 grams of carbohydrates per day. In other words, about 40% of the diet's daily calories come from carbs, whereas the USDA Dietary Guidelines recommend a diet that is 45 to 65% carbohydrates.

The USDA also emphasizes that a healthy eating plan includes grains and dairy products, which are not represented in Optavia's 5 & 1 plan.

There are several popular diet plans that are similar to Optavia, but with key differences that might influence whether they are a good fit for your goals.

SlimFast Diet

When you think of meal replacements, SlimFast probably comes to mind first. While the food and product aspects of SlimFast and Optavia's plans are similar, there are some key differences.

SlimFast's array of meal replacement products is similar in nutrition but you won't find as much variety as with Optavia's plan. However, an attribute of SlimFast is that it does offer meal replacement lines that comply with special diets, such as keto and diabetic weight loss.

If you like the idea of having built-in social support and coaching, that's a key feature of Optavia's plan that you won't find with a SlimFast diet.

Special K Diet

Another popular meal replacement plan is the Special K diet. To follow the two-week "challenge," you'll replace two meals a day with Special K cereal or another Special K product, then eat your usual dinner.

The Special K diet is essentially a "quick-fix" or "crash diet," and is not intended for longer-term use. Optavia's 5 & 1 plan also offers quick weight loss but with a bit more variety than two meals of cereal a day.

With Optavia, you can also transition to the 3 & 3 or 4 & 2 & 1 plans for weight maintenance once you meet your initial goal.

If cost is your main consideration, two weeks' of the Special K diet is certainly a cheaper option than most diet programs including Optavia's.

Do "Quick Fix" Weight Loss Diets Work?

Like Optavia, Nutrisystem is a meal replacement company that sends users pre-made, pre-packaged foods that take the planning and guesswork out of meal prep and planning. However, in contrast to Optavia's "fuelings," Nutrisystem's products more closely resemble typical meals.

Nutrisystem's food choices, such as pizza, sandwiches, and mac and cheese, are intended to stand in for all three meals a day. If the social support aspect of diet programs appeals to you, Nutrisystem also offers support services from on-call counselors.

If you thrive on structure and need to lose weight quickly, the Optavia Diet could be a good fit for you. With its extremely low-calorie eating plans, it's certainly likely to help you shed pounds; however, whether that weight loss will stick once you go off the diet is debatable.

Before you begin any meal replacement diet, carefully consider whether you can realistically follow it, decide how much money you can invest, and determine the degree of hunger and interruption to your social routine you are comfortable with. If you decide to opt for Optavia and succeed with your short-term weight loss goals, make sure you become educated about healthy eating so you can keep the weight off long-term. Also, remember that a calorie-restricted commercial diet is not the only way to slim down. Talk to your healthcare provider or a registered dietitian about simple changes you can make to create a more satisfying nutritious meal plan to help you achieve your goals.

If you're investing the most popular diet plans to lose weight, you'll find the Optimal Weight 5 & 1 plan on your list of programs to consider. But trying to choose the right plan can be tricky and there are many different factors to evaluate.

Dieters on the OPTAVIA 5 & 1 Plan eat five commercially prepared meal replacements each day plus one Lean
& Green meal that you prepare yourself. Meal replacements are familiar foods like mashed potatoes, brownies, pasta, muffins, or soups that have been engineered to provide more protein, less carbohydrate, and limited fat.

Taste

Success on the 5 & 1 Plan requires that you eat a lot of OPTAVIA food. There are plenty of options to choose from and I took a week to sample several popular items. The verdict?

While the foods don't necessarily taste like their "real-world" counterparts, the food didn't taste bad.

For example, the brownie was warm and somewhat chocolatey but didn't necessarily offer the satisfaction of a regular brownie. Mashed potatoes were bland but the consistency was good and I found them modestly satisfying. If you don't have time to cook your own Lean & Green meal (a combination of lean protein and non-starchy vegetables) you can rely on an OPTAVIA Flavors of Home meal. The microwavable meals do not need to be refrigerated so they are quick and convenient. Choices include Turkey Meatball Marinara, Chicken with Rice and Vegetables, and Chicken Cacciatore.

So, how do they taste? I only tried one (Chicken Cacciatore) and would suggest that dieters opt to cook their own meal.

Coaching and Support

OPTAVIA offers several tools to help guide you through the weight loss process:

Online tools to record data: You can record your meal plans, weight loss, exercise, and measurements online or with the Mobile App. Dieters can use these tools at home, at work, or on-the-go to keep their diet journals up to date. As you progress or when you hit struggles you can review data to make changes as necessary.

Community support: Through the online community, you can connect with other dieters to share tips, get feedback about struggles, share successes, and make new friends. Many times, it is the support of fellow dieters that means the most when you are trying to lose weight.

Physician support: Some dieters gain access to OPTAVIA foods and programs through their physicians. For clients with health considerations, this may be the safest option. Not all physicians, however, are part of the nationwide network. You may have to go outside of your network to find a physician who is.

Health coaches: OPTAVIA offers clients the option to buy foods through agents they call "health coaches." These are not certified health professionals but rather agents who have demonstrated knowledge of the OPTAVIA program and who earn income from selling and promoting the foods.4 While some of the coaches may carry outside credentials, clients should not assume that they have expertise in the fields of health, nutrition, diet, or weight loss.

Cost

119 servings of OPTAVIA food will cost $414.60.*

The minimum total cost for a 12-16 week program might range from $1385.40 (12 weeks) to $1878.15 (16 weeks) for the initial part of the plan.

But there are other costs to consider. Of course, you need to factor in the cost of your home-cooked Lean & Green Meal. Alternatively, if you choose to eat OPTAVIA's Flavors of Home meals, add at least $30 per week. Lastly, as you transition off the plan, you'll still eat OPTAVIA meal replacements for at least 6 weeks. This could add several hundred dollars to your bottom line.

Weight Loss

Every dieter is different and different weight loss plans work for different people. Evaluate these pros and cons of Medifast before you make a final decision about whether this is the best diet for you.

- **Pros**

The benefits of this plan include:

Simplicity: You won't have to keep detailed notes or count calories while you lose weight on OPTAVIA. You simply need to count to five. Foods are exceptionally easy to cook and take a few minutes to prepare.

Convenient: There is no excuse not to stick to this diet. The foods are microwavable and some need no preparation at all. You can easily throw a meal replacement packet or a bar into your purse or briefcase for diet-friendly eating on the go. This would be a good diet for people who have very hectic schedules, travel often or don't have time to cook.

- **Cons**

Possible drawbacks of this diet are:

Food taste: While most of the food wasn't bad, it wasn't great either. Foodies and people who love to cook may suffer on this plan. For this reason, some dieters may struggle to stick to the plan long enough to lose their weight.

Potentially difficult transition: The type of foods offered on the plan may make it difficult to transition off the plan when you've reached your goal. OPTAVIA guides clients through a reasonable transition program where they step down and add real-world foods to their diet. But if dieters grab the high-fat and high-carb real-world counterparts to the foods they've gotten used to (like brownies, mashed potatoes or cheese curls), they may gain weight.

Expense: The OPTAVIA 5 & 1 Plan is not cheap. But most plans that offer convenience tend to be pricey. If you choose to go on the program, make sure that you plan for the total cost of your entire weight loss journey so that you don't quit halfway through because you can't afford it.

Take plenty of time to evaluate this or any diet before you invest your money and time. Ask yourself five important questions to make sure you get a program that fits your lifestyle and your needs.

S tudies haven't shown major problems with OPTAVIA. Side effects might include leg cramps, dizziness or fatigue, headaches, loose skin, hair loss, rashes, gas, diarrhea, bad breath, gallstones or gallbladder disease for those at risk, constipation and (for women) menstrual changes.

The apparent absence of noteworthy risks does not mean OPTAVIA is safe for everyone. Pregnant women and those younger than 13 years old shouldn't be on any program, while teens, nursing mothers, people with gout and others should stick to those programs geared toward them (after clearing it with their doctors, of course). Older, sedentary adults and people who exercise more than 45 minutes a day should avoid the 5&1 Program. People with serious illnesses like cancer, liver disease, kidney disease or an eating disorder shouldn't follow any plan unless their health care providers have cleared them as recovered and stabilized.

If you're on any medications especially warfarin, lithium, diabetes medication or medications for high blood pressure talk to your doctor before starting any of the programs, the company advises.

Is Optavia Diet a heart-healthy diet?

OPTAVIA may possibly be heart healthy, but no more than many other diets. OPTAVIA contends its Fuelings are low in fat and cholesterol, and many contain enough high-quality soy protein to meet the Food and Drug Administration's Heart Health claim.

OPTAVIA represents the community of coaches and lifestyle brand launched in 2017. Previous studies were conducted using some products, not the new OPTAVIA products. While the OPTAVIA products represent a new line, Medifast has advised U.S. News that they have an identical macronutrient profile and as such are interchangeable with the Medifast products. Therefore, we believe these studies are relevant when evaluating this diet.

In the 2017 Medifast-sponsored study in the journal Nutrition and Diabetes, participants significantly reduced their blood pressure. A study found that overweight and obese participants following the 4&2&1 Plan significantly improved their blood pressure. In the 2010 Nutrition Journal study described in the weight-loss section, researchers reported declines in blood pressure, pulse rate and blood levels of C-reactive protein, a marker of inflammation that may predict heart disease risk, in the Medifast and control groups at week 40. The study also reported on waist size and amount of abdominal fat, which are thought to be indicators of heart disease risk. At week 40, Medifast dieters had lost an average of about 4 inches around the waist, the control group about 1 1/2 inches. The abdominal "fat rating" for both groups had decreased as well, but the Medifast group performed slightly better. At week 40, total cholesterol was not significantly lower for the Medifast group but had dropped appreciably for the control group. Neither group showed improved levels of triglycerides, a fatty substance that in excess has been linked to heart disease, at 40 weeks.

In the Diabetes Educator study, the Medifast dieters had significantly higher good HDL cholesterol and lower systolic blood pressure after 86 weeks, but neither change was significant when compared to the control group.

Optavia Meal Plan

- **Breakfast Serving Size**

¾   cup ready-to-eat unsweetened cereal

1 cup skim or low-fat milk 1 Starch

1 Dairy

- **Mid-Morning Fueling**

Optimal Health Strawberry Yogurt Bar 1 Optimal Health Fueling

- **Lunch**

½   cup cooked cauliflower

3 oz. grilled chicken ¾ cup low-fat yogurt 1 Vegetable

1 Protein

1 Dairy

- **Mid-Afternoon Fueling**

Optimal Health Strawberry Banana Smoothie 1 Optimal Health Fueling

- **Dinner**

2 cups raw spinach

1 cup total diced tomatoes, cucumbers, and mushrooms

3 oz. baked yellowfin tuna

2 Tbsp low-fat salad dressing

1 small apple

1 Protein

1 Fat

1 Fruit

1. **GARLIC CHICKEN WITH ZOODLES**

This creamy garlic chicken is one of our favorite lean and green recipes! It's colorful and packed full of flavor without the guilt!

Prep Time: 15 mins

Cook Time: 15 mins

Total Time: 30 mins

INGREDIENTS

1 1/2 lbs boneless skinless chicken breasts

1 T olive oil

1 C low fat plain greek yogurt

1/2 C chicken broth

1/2 tsp garlic powder

1/2 tsp italian seasoning

1/4 C parmesan cheese

1 C spinach, chopped

3-6 slices sun dried tomatoes

1 T chopped garlic

1 1/2 C zucchini cut into thin noodles

INSTRUCTIONS

HOW TO COOK THE CHICKEN

Heat the oil in a large skillet on medium.

Using paper towels, pat the chicken breast dry, sprinkle with salt and pepper for taste and place in hot oil.

Cook on medium high for for 3-5 minutes on each side or until brown on each side and until no longer pink in center.

Remove chicken and set aside on a plate.

Add the yogurt, chicken broth, garlic powder, Italian seasoning, and parmesan cheese into the large skillet.

Whisk over medium high heat until it starts to thicken.

Add the spinach and sun dried tomatoes.

Simmer until the spinach starts to wilt.

Add the chicken back to the pan and serve over zucchini noodles.

HOW TO COOK THE ZOODLES

Preheat oven to 350 degrees F.

Using vegetable spiraler, cut zucchini into the shape of spiral noodles.

Place parchment paper on a large baking sheet. Spread and arrange zoodles and toss with sea salt. Be sure to spread them thin so they don't stick together.

Bake for 15 min for al dente. Add a couple minutes if you want them softer.

Serve right away.

2.   **Optavia Biscuit Pizza Ingredients**

1 sachet Optavia Buttermilk Cheddar and Herb Biscuit

2 Tbsp water

1 Tbsp tomato sauce

1 Tbsp low fat shredded cheese

Instructions

Preheat oven or toaster to 350 degrees F.

Stir together biscuit and water and spread into a thin circle on parchment paper and cook for 10 minutes.

Add tomato sauce then shredded cheese and bake for a few more minutes, until the cheese has melted.

3. **Lean and Green**

Prep: 10 mins

Total: 10 mins

Servings: 1

Ingredient

1 cup fresh spinach

1 banana

½ green apple
4 hulled strawberries

4 (1 inch) pieces frozen mango

⅓ Cup whole milk

1 scoop vanilla protein powder (Optional)

1 teaspoon honey

Directions

Blend spinach, banana, apple, strawberries, mango, milk, protein powder, and honey together in a blender until smooth.

4. **Medifast Chicken Stir Fry**

Minutes to Prepare: 10

Minutes to Cook: 10

Number of Servings: 2

Ingredients

12 oz skinless, boneless chicken breast

1 cup chopped red bell pepper

1 cup chopped green bell pepper

8 oz (1 cup) broccoli slaw

1/2 cup chicken broth

2 tbs low sodium no carb soy sauce

1 tsp crushed red pepper

Directions

Sautee peppers and broccoli slaw in chicken broth. Add soy sauce, add chicken and red pepper. Cook for a few more minutes until peppers are tender.

5.   **OPTAVIA Mini Mac In A Bowl**

INGREDIENTS

2 Tablespoons yellow or white onion; diced
5 ounces 95-97% Lean Ground Beef

2 Tablespoons Wish-Bone Light Thousand Island dressing

1/8 teaspoon White Vinegar

1/8 teaspoon Onion Powder

3 cups Romaine Lettuce; shredded

2 Tablespooons Reduced-Fat Cheddar Cheese; shredded

1 ounce Dill Pickle Slices

1 teaspoon sesame seeds

Cooking Spray

INSTRUCTIONS

1. Heat a small, lightly greased skillet over medium-high heat. Add the onion & cook until fragrant, about 2-3 minutes. Add the beef and cook until fully browned.

2. Meanwhile, mix together the dressing, vinegar and onion powder.

3. To assemble: Top lettuce with the ground beef and sprinkle with cheese. Top with pickle slices. Drizzle with sauce, and sprinkle with sesame seeds.

6.   **Avocado Citrus Shrimp Salad**

YIELDS 2 Servings

PREP TIME: 25 mins

COOK TIME: 5 mins

TOTAL TIME: 30 mins

INGREDIENTS

½   lb wild caught shrimp (uncooked)

1 avocado

1 head green leaf lettuce (or any other mild lettuce)

2 tbsp olive oil (try The Crescent Olive's Lime Extra Virgin Olive Oil!)

Sea salt, pepper, cayenne, cumin, garlic powder, onion powder

Juice of lemon or lime

Microgreens (optional)

DIRECTION

Prepare the lettuce:

Wash, dry, and chop lettuce. Arrange on 2 plates and set aside.

Prepare the Shrimp:

Remove tails from shrimp and place in strainer to remove excess liquid.

Transfer to mixing bowl and combine with spices. Toss gently to coat evenly.

Heat 1 tbsp. olive oil in a skillet over medium-low heat.

Cook shrimp for 2-3 minutes on one side, flip and cook for 1-2 minutes on the second side. Cover, turn off heat, and let shrimp continue to cook through for a few more minutes.

Prepare the Avocado:

Slice avocado in half around the pit. On each side, score the flesh to create cubes of avocado. Invert skin to release avocado cubes. Place on top of lettuce.

Prepare the Dressing:

In a small bowl, combine 2 tbsp. olive oil, juice of 1/2 lemon or lime, salt and pepper. Whisk together until combined.

Put it all together:

Arrange cooked shrimp on top of lettuce.

Using a spoon, distribute dressing over salads.

Top with more of the spices that were used to season the shrimp.

Top with microgreens (if using) and serve immediately!

The olive oil and lemon juice help your body to assimilate and absorb the fat soluble nutrients in the green lettuce, the citrus prevents the avocado from browning, and all ingredients compliment each other for a complete meal!

7.   **BROCCOLI TACO BOWL**

This Broccoli Taco Bowl is Gluten Free and helps you stay on track with your weight loss goals!

PREP TIME: 2 mins

COOK TIME: 10 mins

TOTAL TIME: 12 mins

SERVINGS 1

INGREDIENTS

4- oz lean ground hamburger

1- oz shredded cheddar cheese

1 1/4 cup broccoli, cut into bite sized pieces

1/4 cup Rotel tomatoes

1/4 teaspoon garlic powder

1/4 teaspoon onion powder

1/4 teaspoon salt, divided

Pinch of red pepper flakes

2 tablespoons low sodium chicken stock

DIRECTIONS

Put your broccoli in a bowl with your chicken stock and cover with plastic wrap. Put in the microwave for 4 minutes, or until tender and cooked.

In a large skillet brown your hamburger and drain the grease if needed when it's done.

Add your Rotel tomatoes, garlic powder, onion powder, salt, and red pepper flakes and stir well.

When your broccoli is finished cooking then add it to your skillet and toss with the hamburger mixture.
Add everything to a bowl and top with your shredded cheddar cheese.

8. **Mac & Cheese: The Lean Green**

COOK TIME: 30 minutes

Ingredients

1 lb small shell pasta (455 g)

3 ½ cups whole milk (840 mL)

8 tablespoons unsalted butter

2 cups shredded american cheese (200 g)

2 teaspoons kosher salt

½ teaspoon ground black pepper

2 cups broccoli floret (300 g), steamed

½ cup shredded parmesan cheese (55 g)

Preparation

In a large pot over medium heat, combine the pasta and milk. Bring the milk to a simmer and cook until the pasta is tender, 8–10 minutes.

Once the pasta is cooked, remove the pan from the heat and add the butter, American cheese, salt, and pepper.
Stir until fully combined. Fold in the broccoli.

Divide between serving bowls and top with the Parmesan cheese.

Enjoy!

9. **OPTAVIA CLOUD BREAD**

Yields: 3 Servings

INGREDIENTS

1/16 teaspoon Cream of Tartar

3 Eggs

1/2 cup Fat-Free 0% Plain Greek Yogurt

1 packet sweetener

DIRECTION

At least 1/2 hour before making, put the whisk attachment and Kitchen Aid Bowl in the freezer.

Preheat oven to 300 degrees. Get the bowl & whisk attachment out of the Freezer. Separate the eggs.

Put the whites in the Kitchen Aid Bowl and the yolks in a different medium-sized bowl. In the medium-sized bowl with the yolks, mix in the Greek Yogurt and sweetener. In the bowl with the egg whites, add in the cream of tartar.

Beat this mixture until the egg whites form stiff peaks. Take the egg yolk mixture and gently fold it into the egg whites.

Do not over-stir.

Put parchment paper on a baking tray.

Spray with cooking spray.

Scoop out 6 equally-sized "blobs" of the "dough" onto the parchment paper. Bake 25-35 minutes (check at 25 minutes.

In some ovens, they are done at this point).

They will get brownish on the top and crackled. Most people prefer them cold vs warm. Many people like to re-heat in a toaster or toast oven to get them somewhat crispy.

10.   **Optavia Pizza Hack**

Prep Time: 10 mins

Cook Time: 16 mins

Servings: 1

Equipment

Parchment Paper

2 Baking sheets

Saute pan

Ingredients

Pizza Crust

1 packet Garlic Smashed Potato Packet 1 Fueling

2 Egg Whites* 1/7 Leanest

1 tsp Baking Powder** 2 Condiments

Pizza Toppings

1/4 cup Pizza Sauce*** 1 Green

1/2 cup Sliced white mushrooms 1 Green

3 oz Reduced Fat Shredded Mozzarella 3/4 Lean

1.5 oz Ground Beef 1/4 Leaner

2 Black Olives sliced 1/4 Fat

Instructions

Bake Crust

Preheat Oven to 400 degrees.

Mix together the garlic potato packet and baking powder.

Add egg whites and stir until combined.

Pour batter onto parchment paper lined baking sheet.

Top with another piece of parchment paper and spread out the batter to a 1/8 of an inch circle.

Top with second baking sheet so the crust is sandwiched between the two sheets.
 Bake for 8 minutes or until crust is golden brown.

Add Toppings to Pizza

While crust is baking, brown ground beef in a saute pan, wash the mushrooms, and measure your toppings.

When crust is done, pull out of oven put aside top baking sheet and peel back the top layer of parchment paper.

Be careful as paper might stick at this step.

Layer pizza sauce, shredded cheese, and toppings.

Bake for another 8 minutes. When the pizza is ready it should slide right off the parchment paper and easily transfer to a plate.

11. **Chicken Pesto Pasta**

This lightened up Lean Green Chicken Pesto Pasta tastes like spring in a bite. A quick low-fat pesto, tossed with chickpea pasta, chicken, and fresh mozzarella, you will get yourself a flavorful and nutritious meal in under 30 minutes!

Makes: 5 servings (just over 8 cups)

Prep Time: 15 minutes

Total Time: 30 minutes

Ingredients

Kale Pesto

3 cups (48g) raw kale (stems removed)

2 cup (12g) fresh basil

2 tablespoons (28g) olive oil

3 tablespoons lemon juice

3 garlic cloves

¼   teaspoon salt

Pasta Salad

2 cups (280g) cooked chicken breast (diced)

6 oz (176g) uncooked "Barilla" rotini chickpea pasta

1 cup (20g) arugula or baby spinach

3oz (84g) "Bel Gioioso" fresh mozzarella (diced)

Optional: additional basil leaves or red pepper flakes for garnish
Instructions

24

Make the pesto by adding the kale, basil, olive oil, garlic cloves, lemon juice, and salt to a food processor. Blend until smooth. Season to taste with additional salt and pepper.

Cook pasta according to package directions. Strain, reserving ¼ cup cooking liquid. In a large bowl, mix together the cooked pasta, diced chicken, pesto, arugula or spinach, reserved pasta liquid, and mozzarella and toss until combined. Sprinkle with extra chopped basil or red pepper flakes (if desired).

Serve chilled or warm. This pasta salad is delicious on its own, as a salad mix-in, or as a side! Store leftovers in an airtight container in the refrigerator for 3-5 days. Enjoy!

12.   **Crockpot Chili**

This lean and Green Crock Pot Chili Recipe is a yummy lightened up Green Chili recipe made in the slow cooker and is only 241 calories per serving!

Prep Time: 10 minutes

Cook Time: 5 hours

Total Time: 5 hours 10 minutes

Ingredients

1 pound boneless skinless chicken breasts cut into 3/4 inch pieces

1/2 cup chopped onions

2 tsp Ground Cumin

1 to 2 tsp garlic

1/2 tsp chili powder

Salt and pepper (about 1/4 tsp each)

2 cans of fat free chicken broth

1 can of green enchilada sauce (or 1 1/2 cup of salsa verde)

8 6-inch corn tortillas broken into very small pieces (divided)

3/4 cup of corn

2 cans of beans, drained and rinsed (Black or pinto)

1 tsp cornstarch

1/2 evaporated milk or (1/3 cup of dry milk and 1/2 cup water)

Optional toppings:

2 tsp snipped fresh cilantro

Sour cream

Shredded Cheese

Instructions

Add chicken, chopped onion, chicken broth, enchilada sauce, spices and half of the broken up corn tortillas to the crock-pot and mix everything together.

Cook on low for 4 hours.

Once the chili has cooked for 4 hours, add the corn, beans, and the rest of the broken up tortillas to the crock pot.

Stir the cornstarch into the evaporated milk (or dry milk/water) until completely dissolved.

Mix cornstarch Mixture into the chili.

Cook on low for 1 more hour.

Serve and then top with optional sour cream, shredded cheese and cilantro.

Enjoy!

13.   Green Beans, Ground Turkey and Rice

This ground turkey and rice recipe gets a major upgrade by adding crispy green beans and a bit of sesame oil for some extra flavor.

Prep Time: 15 minutes

Cook Time: 13 minutes

Total Time: 28 minutes

4 Servings

Ingredients

1 Tbsp. + 1 tsp. sesame oil

1 lb. 93% lean ground turkey raw

5 cups green beans ends trimmed

Sea salt (or Himalayan salt) and

ground black pepper to taste;

optional 1⅓ cups brown rice

cooked

Instructions

Heat oil in large skillet over medium-high heat.

Add turkey; cook, stirring frequently, for 4 to 6 minutes, or until browned and no longer pink.

Add green beans; cook, covered, stirring occasionally, for 4 to 6 minutes, or until green beans are tender crisp.

Season with salt and pepper (if desired); mix well.

Serve each portion over ⅓ cup rice.

14.   LEAN AND GREEN GARLIC CHICKEN WITH ZOODLES

This creamy garlic chicken is one of our favorite lean and green recipes! It's colorful and packed full of flavor without the guilt!

Prep Time: 15 mins

Cook Time: 15 mins

Total Time: 30 mins

INGREDIENTS

1 1/2 lbs boneless skinless chicken breasts

1 T olive oil

1 C low fat plain greek yogurt

1/2 C chicken broth

1/2 tsp garlic powder

1/2 tsp italian seasoning

1/4 C parmesan cheese

1 C spinach, chopped

3-6 slices sun dried tomatoes

1 T chopped garlic

1 1/2 C zucchini cut into thin noodles

INSTRUCTIONS

HOW TO COOK THE CHICKEN

Heat the oil in a large skillet on medium.

Using paper towels, pat the chicken breast dry, sprinkle with salt and pepper for taste and place in hot oil.

Cook on medium high for 3-5 minutes on each side or until brown on each side and until no longer pink in center.

Remove chicken and set aside on a plate.

Add the yogurt, chicken broth, garlic powder, Italian seasoning, and parmesan cheese into the large skillet.

Whisk over medium high heat until it starts to thicken.

Add the spinach and sun dried tomatoes.

Simmer until the spinach starts to wilt.

Add the chicken back to the pan and serve over zucchini noodles.

HOW TO COOK THE ZOODLES

Preheat oven to 350 degrees F.

Using vegetable spiraler, cut zucchini into the shape of spiral noodles.

Place parchment paper on a large baking sheet. Spread and arrange zoodles and toss with sea salt. Be sure to spread them thin so they don't stick together.

Bake for 15 min for al dente. Add a couple minutes if you want them softer.

Serve right away.

15.   **BBQ Turkey Burgers**

Fire up the grill for BBQ Turkey Burgers tonight! BBQ Turkey Burgers are ultra-moist and tasty, making them a great alternative to traditional high-fat beef patties. Sweet onion is a tasty contradiction to tangy BBQ sauce. Try it with grilled pineapple too.

Yield: Makes 4 burgers (serving size: 1 bbq turkey burger)

Ingredients

1 pound ground dark-meat turkey

1 garlic clove, minced

1/2 teaspoon paprika

1/4 teaspoon ground cumin

Pinch of kosher salt

1/4 teaspoon freshly ground black pepper

4 slices sweet onion, grilled

1/4 cup barbecue sauce

4 (1.6-oz) sesame seed buns, toasted

Directions

In medium bowl, gently mix together turkey, garlic, paprika, and cumin.

Form turkey into 4 (4-inch) patties; season with salt and pepper.

Heat grill to medium-high; cook, turning once, until burgers are just cooked through (about 7 minutes per side).

Serve with desired toppings and buns.

16. **Energy-Revving Quinoa**

This meatless meal of Energy-Revving Quinoa keeps you

energized between meals or after a workout. Yield: Makes 1

serving (serving size: 1 1/2 cups)

Ingredients

1 cup cooked quinoa

1/3 cup canned low-sodium black beans, drained and rinsed

1 small tomato, chopped

1 scallion, sliced

1 teaspoon olive oil

1 teaspoon fresh lemon juice

Pinch of salt

Pinch of freshly ground black pepper

Directions

In a medium bowl, gently toss all ingredients to combine.

17. **Steakhouse Salad**

Break out this recipe for the hard-core carnivores in your life. It's everything they (and you) love about a steakhouse meal, succulent beef, creamy spinach, and roasted potatoes in salad form. Mushrooms and cherry tomatoes bump up the veg factor, and a light yet full-flavored blue cheese dressing ties it all together.

Active: 25 mins

Total: 25 mins

Yield: Serves 4

Ingredients

10 ounces (4 to 5 small) red potatoes, quartered

2 tablespoons canola oil, divided

1 teaspoon black pepper, divided

1/2 teaspoon kosher salt, divided

1 (8-oz.) beef tenderloin filet

8 ounces cremini mushrooms, quartered

3 garlic cloves, chopped (about 1 1/2 Tbsp.)

1 tablespoon lower-sodium Worcestershire sauce

2 cups cherry tomatoes

1/3 cup low-fat buttermilk

1 tablespoon apple cider vinegar

3 ounces blue cheese, crumbled (about 3/4 cup), divided

8 cups fresh baby spinach (about 6 oz.)

Directions

Preheat oven to 400°F. Toss potatoes with 1 tablespoon of the oil and 1/4 teaspoon each of the pepper and salt on a rimmed baking sheet. Roast potatoes until golden and tender, about 20 minutes, stirring halfway through baking.

Meanwhile, heat remaining 1 tablespoon oil in a heavy skillet over medium-high. Sprinkle beef with 1/4 teaspoon of the pepper and remaining 1/4 teaspoon salt. Sear beef until browned on all sides and a thermometer registers 130°F to 135°F (for medium-rare), about 3 minutes per side, or to desired degree of doneness. Transfer beef to a plate; let rest 5 minutes before slicing.

Return skillet to medium-high. Add mushrooms and garlic, and cook, stirring often, until browned, 2 to 3 minutes. Stir in 2 tablespoons water and Worcestershire, and cook 1 minute. Remove mushroom mixture. Add

31

tomatoes to skillet; cook, stirring occasionally, until blistered, about 4 minutes. Remove from heat.

Stir together buttermilk, vinegar, 1/2 cup of the blue cheese, and remaining 1/2 teaspoon pepper in a large bowl.
Toss spinach in butter milk mixture.

Serve spinach topped with potatoes, beef, mushroom mixture, and tomatoes; sprinkle with remaining 1/4 cup blue cheese.

18. **Salmon Noodle Bowl**

Omega-3s in salmon and other fatty fish help build more muscle, and more muscle means more calories burned.

Prep: 8 mins

Cook: 20 mins

Total: 28 mins

Yield: Makes 2 servings (serving size: 2 1/4 cups)

Ingredients

4 ounces soba buckwheat noodles or whole-wheat spaghetti

5 ounces asparagus, cut in thirds

Cooking spray
1 (6-oz) salmon fillet, skin off, cut into 8 pieces

1 tablespoon toasted sesame oil

Zest and juice of 1-2 limes (3 TBSP juice)

1/4 teaspoon kosher salt

1/4 teaspoon fresh pepper

4 ounces cucumber, skin on, cut into medium pieces

1/2 small avocado, cut into bite-size pieces

Directions

Cook the noodles in boiling water until soft (about 6 minutes for soba, 8 for spaghetti). Transfer with tongs to a strainer. Add asparagus to same boiling water. Cook until al dente (about 2 minutes); rinse under cold water.

Heat a grill pan or skillet over medium-high heat. Coat lightly with cooking spray. Cook the salmon until cooked through, turning pieces (about 2-3 minutes per side). Reserve.

Make the vinaigrette: Whisk together sesame oil, lime zest and juice, and salt and pepper in a small bowl.
Combine the noodles, asparagus, and vinaigrette in a medium serving bowl.

Add the cucumber and avocado; toss to coat. Just before serving, add salmon. Serve warm or at room temperature, or make up to 4 hours ahead and keep refrigerated in an airtight container.

19. Cauliflower and Mushroom Tacos

Serve these as a vegetarian meal, or with meat-based tacos to mix things up.

Active: 25 mins

Total: 25 mins

Yield: Serves 4

Ingredients

1 cup very thinly sliced red onion

1/4 cup red wine vinegar

1 cup dark Mexican beer (such as Negra Modelo)

1 tablespoon honey

2 tablespoons canola oil

12 ounces cauliflower florets (from 1 head)

6 ounces cremini mushrooms, quartered
1 teaspoon kosher salt

1 teaspoon ground cumin

1/2 teaspoon ancho chile powder

1/4 cup chopped fresh cilantro

8 (6-in.) corn tortillas, warmed

Cotija cheese, pico de gallo, and diced avocado, for garnish

Lime wedges, for serving

Directions

Toss together onion and vinegar in a microwavable dish. Microwave on High for 1 minute; set aside.

Bring beer to a boil in a small saucepan over high; cook until reduced to ½ cup, about 5 minutes. Stir in honey.

Heat oil in a large skillet over high. Add cauliflower and mushrooms. Cook, stirring often, until caramelized and softened, 6 to 8 minutes. Add salt, cumin, and chile powder; cook, stirring often, until fragrant, about 1 minute. Add beer mixture and cilantro; cook, stirring occasionally, until vegetables are tender, about 2 minutes.

Divide vegetable mixture among tortillas. Gently stir onion mixture, and drain any liquid. Top tacos with pickled onion, and garnish with Cotija, pico de gallo, and avocado, if desired. Serve with lime wedges.

20.   Black Bean and Chicken Chilaquiles

Total: 45 mins

Yield: 6 servings

Ingredients

Cooking spray

1 cup thinly sliced onion

5 garlic cloves, minced

2 cups shredded cooked chicken breast

1 (15-ounce) can black beans, rinsed and drained

1 cup fat-free, less-sodium chicken broth

1 (7 3/4-ounce) can salsa de chile fresco (such as El Pato)

15 (6-inch) corn tortillas, cut into 1-inch strips

1 cup shredded queso blanco (about 4 ounces)

Directions

Preheat oven to 450°. Heat a large nonstick skillet over medium-high heat. Coat pan with cooking spray. Add
onion; sauté 5 minutes or until lightly browned. Add garlic; sauté 1 minute. Add chicken; cook 30 seconds. Transfer mixture to a medium bowl; stir in beans. Add broth and salsa to pan; bring to a boil. Reduce heat, and simmer 5 minutes, stirring occasionally. Set aside.

Place half of tortilla strips in bottom of an 11 x 7-inch baking dish coated with cooking spray. Layer half of chicken mixture over tortillas; top with remaining tortillas and chicken mixture. Pour broth mixture evenly over chicken mixture. Sprinkle with cheese. Bake at 450° for 10 minutes or until tortillas are lightly browned and cheese is melted.

21.   **Cioppino**

This technique takes the intimidation out of cooking shellfish. As long as you add each type at its indicated time instead of all at once, you'll end up with delicate, perfectly cooked clams, scallops, shrimp, and mussels. And the flavor of this stew is so rich and deep, you'd never guess it all comes together in about half an hour. This technique takes the intimidation out of cooking shellfish. As long as you add each type at its indicated time instead of all at once, you'll end up with delicate, perfectly cooked clams, scallops, shrimp, and mussels. And the flavor of this stew is so rich and deep, you'd never guess it all comes together in about half an hour.

Active: 35 mins

Total: 35 mins

Yield: Serves 4

Ingredients

1 tablespoon extra-virgin olive oil

1 small yellow onion, sliced

1 small fennel bulb, trimmed and sliced

6 garlic cloves, sliced

1 cup dry white wine

1/4 cup seafood stock

1/4 cup chopped fresh basil, plus more for garnish

1/2 teaspoon crushed red pepper

1 (28-oz.) can no-salt-added whole tomatoes, drained

12 littleneck clams, scrubbed (about 6 oz.)

8 sea scallops (about 8 oz.)

1/2 teaspoon kosher salt

1/2 teaspoon black pepper

8 large peeled and deveined raw shrimp (about 8 oz.)

12 mussels, scrubbed and debearded (about 6 oz.)
2 tablespoon fresh lemon juice

Directions

Heat oil in a large Dutch oven over medium-high; swirl to coat. Add onion and fennel; cook, stirring often, 1 minute. Add garlic; reduce heat to medium, cover, and cook, stirring occasionally, until vegetables are tender, about 8 minutes. Stir in wine, stock, basil, red pepper, and tomatoes; increase heat to medium-high, cover, and bring to a boil. Reduce heat to medium-low, and simmer 10 minutes.

Increase heat to medium-high. Add clams to skillet; cover and cook 2 minutes. Sprinkle scallops with salt and pepper. Add scallops; cover and cook 2 minutes. Add shrimp and mussels; cover and cook until clams and mussels open, about 4 minutes. Discard any unopened shells. Gently stir in lemon juice, and, if desired, sprinkle with basil.

22.   Harissa Shakshuka With Spinach & Chickpeas

Bring big flavor to the table, and your diabetic-friendly diet, with this Israeli-inspired dish. Cooking the eggs sunny-side up in a rich tomato sauce imbues them with umami, and a light crumble of feta adds a salty pop to every bite.

Active: 30 mins

Total: 30 mins

Yield: Serves 6

Ingredients

1 tablespoon olive oil

1 cup sliced yellow onion

1 cup chopped red bell pepper

1 cup chopped yellow bell pepper

2 cups lower-sodium marinara sauce

2 tablespoons mild or hot harissa

1 tablespoon chopped fresh oregano

1/2 teaspoon kosher salt

1 (15-oz.) can no-salt-added chickpeas, drained and rinsed

1 (6-oz.) pkg. fresh baby spinach (about 9 cups

6 large eggs

2 ounces feta cheese, crumbled (about ½ cup)

2 tablespoons fresh lemon juice (from one lemon)

Fresh flat-leaf parsley, for garnish

Directions

Heat oil in a large skillet over medium-high. Add onion and bell peppers, and cook, stirring often, until softened, 6 to 8 minutes. Stir in marinara, harissa, oregano, salt, chickpeas, and spinach. Cook, stirring occasionally, until spinach wilts, about 3 minutes.

Make 6 shallow wells in mixture; crack 1 egg into each well. Cover, reduce heat to medium-low, and cook until whites are cooked but yolks are still runny, about 5 minutes.

Remove from heat; sprinkle mixture with feta and lemon juice, and garnish with parsley.

23.   **Italian Garbanzo Salad**

This can be served as a first course or antipasti with Italian food, or as a side to grilled chicken. It's even better the next day over salad greens.

Yield: 8 servings (serving size: about 1 cup)

Ingredients

3 cups finely chopped fennel bulb

2 cups chopped tomato

1 3/4 cups finely chopped red onion

1 cup chopped fresh basil

1/3 cup balsamic vinegar

1 tablespoon olive oil

1 teaspoon freshly ground black pepper

1/4 teaspoon salt

4 garlic cloves, minced

2 (15 1/2-ounce) cans chickpeas (garbanzo beans), rinsed and drained

1/2 cup (2 ounces) crumbled feta cheese

Directions

Combine all ingredients except the cheese in a bowl; toss well. Let stand 30 minutes; sprinkle with cheese.

24. Poached Salmon With Yogurt-Tarragon Sauce

You don't have to worry about drying out fish when it's cooking in liquid! This preparation is so delicate and subtle you can taste the aromatics that are in the cooking liquid, but it doesn't take anything away from the flavor of the salmon. Remember that you're poaching, not boiling: The liquid should be below the boiling point or the fish can get rubbery.

Active: 15 mins
 Total: 45 mins

Yield: Serves 4

Ingredients

2 lemons, halved, plus 1 Tbsp. fresh lemon juice

1 cup dry white wine

1 tablespoon whole black peppercorns

2 bay leaves

1/4 cup thinly sliced shallot

1 tablespoon plus ¾ tsp. kosher salt

4 (6-oz.) skinless salmon fillets (1 to 1½ in. thick)

3/4 cup plain whole-milk yogurt

2 tablespoon chopped fresh tarragon, plus more for garnish

1/4 teaspoon black pepper

Directions

Squeeze lemon halves into a high-sided sauté pan or Dutch oven, then add squeezed lemon halves to pan. Add 4 cups water, wine, peppercorns, bay leaves, shallots, and 1 tablespoon of the salt. Bring to a boil over medium-high; cover, reduce heat to medium-low, and simmer 10 minutes. (Adjust heat if needed to make sure liquid is barely steaming with a temperature of about 145°F.)

Add salmon to pan, cover, and cook until a thermometer inserted in fish registers 125°F to 130°F, 10 to 12 minutes. Transfer salmon to a large plate lined with paper towels. Remove and discard any whole peppercorns or bay leaves clinging to fish. Sprinkle fish with ½ teaspoon of the salt. (To serve salmon cold, chill in the refrigerator 30 minutes.)

Stir together yogurt, tarragon, lemon juice, pepper, and remaining ¼ teaspoon salt. If desired, sprinkle fillets with chopped tarragon. Serve with sauce.

25. **Spinach-Quinoa Breakfast Salad With Berries And Granola**

Berries, granola, yogurt and spinach? Trust us. All the makings of your morning parfait create an unexpected dish with pleasing crunch and pretty pops of color.

Active: 10 mins

Total: 10 mins

Yield: Serves 2
Ingredients

2 teaspoon apple cider vinegar

1 teaspoon pure maple syrup

1/4 teaspoon Dijon mustard

1/4 teaspoon kosher salt

1 tablespoon olive oil

1 (7-oz.) container plain Greek yogurt

3 ounces baby spinach (about 3 cups)

2/3 cup cooked quinoa

2/3 cup quartered fresh strawberries (4 oz.)

1/2 cup fresh blueberries

1/2 cup store-bought almond granola

Directions

Whisk together vinegar, maple syrup, mustard, and salt in a small bowl. Slowly drizzle in oil, whisking constantly, until fully emulsified.

Spread yogurt evenly on 2 plates. Toss together spinach, quinoa, strawberries, blueberries, and half of the dressing in a medium bowl. Divide salad between plates, on top of yogurt. Drizzle with remaining dressing, and sprinkle with granola.

26.   **Crisp Chickpea Slaw**

You need only a little dressing for the slaw because the cabbage releases moisture as it sits. You need only a little dressing for the slaw because the cabbage releases moisture as it sits.

Prep: 10 mins

Total: 10 mins

Yield: Makes 2 servings (serving size: 3 1/2 cups)

Ingredients

1/4 cup fat-free plain yogurt

1 tablespoon cider vinegar

1 tablespoon water

1/4 teaspoon kosher salt

Freshly ground black pepper
1 (15-oz) can low-sodium chickpeas, rinsed and drained

2 1/2 cups sliced packed green cabbage

2 stalks celery, thinly sliced

2 carrots, peeled with a vegetable peeler into strips or thinly sliced, or 2 cups shredded carrots

2 tablespoons sesame seeds, toasted

Directions

In a medium bowl, stir together the yogurt, vinegar, water, salt, and pepper to taste. Add the chickpeas, cabbage, celery, and carrots; toss to combine. Sprinkle with sesame seeds.

Transfer slaw to a plastic food-storage bag or 2 portable containers. Refrigerate at least 4 hours before serving; slaw keeps up to 3 days.

27.   **Egg and Rice Salad to Go**

Any hearty brown rice or brown-rice blend works well in this salad. Great use for leftovers: Any hearty brown rice or brown-rice blend works well in this salad.

Prep: 10 mins

Total: 10 mins

Yield: Makes 1 serving (serving size: about 2.5 cups)
Ingredients

1/2 cup cooked brown rice

1 cup cooked green beans, roughly chopped (3 oz)

1 ripe plum, thinly sliced (3 oz)

2 tablespoons (1/2 oz) chopped walnuts

1 hard-cooked egg, sliced

1 teaspoon sesame oil

2 tablespoons fresh lime juice

1/4 teaspoon kosher salt

Freshly ground black pepper, to taste

Directions

Combine rice, beans, plum, walnuts, and egg in a portable container.

Drizzle with sesame oil, lime juice, salt, and pepper; toss gently to combine. Refrigerate up to 2 days.

28.   **Asian Rice Noodle Salad**

Bonus meal: If you have leftover coleslaw mix, sauté it with a little garlic and ginger and add a protein for a faster-than-takeout mu shu.

Active: 15 mins

Total: 20 mins

Yield: 6 as a side dish

Ingredients

1 Asian brown rice (whole-grain) noodles

1/4 cup low-sodium soy sauce

1 tablespoon rice vinegar

2 tablespoons fresh lime juice
2 teaspoons honey

2 teaspoons toasted sesame oil

1 teaspoon minced fresh ginger

1 clove garlic, minced

3/4 cup fresh cilantro leaves, chopped

3/4 cup chopped salted, dry-roasted peanuts or cashews

2 1/2 cups coleslaw mix

Red pepper flakes, optional

Directions

Cook noodles according to package directions. Drain and transfer to a large bowl to cool. Cut noodles up a bit with kitchen shears or a knife to make them easier to toss.

Whisk together soy sauce, vinegar, lime juice, honey, sesame oil, ginger, and garlic in a small bowl.

Add sauce, cilantro, peanuts, and coleslaw mix to bowl with noodles and toss until well combined. Sprinkle with red pepper flakes to taste, if desired. Serve at room temperature or refrigerate for later.

29.   Chard And Mushroom Butternut Noodles

Enjoying more veggies is probably the No. 1 thing you can do to boost your overall health. While these nutritional superstars can help fend off cancer and other chronic diseases, they can also minimize the effects of aging and contribute to shiny hair and glowing skin. See? Veggies are a win-win! They're also irresistibly delicious, especially when served like "pasta" topped with a hazelnut gremolata for depth of flavor and Parmesan cheese for a hit of umami.

Active: 30 mins

Total: 30 mins

Yield: Serves 4

Ingredients

8 cups spiralized butternut squash (1¼ lb.)

3 tablespoons olive oil, divided

2 tablespoons chopped roasted hazelnuts

1 teaspoon lemon zest, plus 2 Tbsp. fresh juice, divided

2 ounces Parmesan cheese, finely shredded (about ¾ cup), divided

2 teaspoons fresh thyme leaves, divided

1 pound sliced fresh cremini mushrooms

8 cups chopped fresh Swiss chard (from 1 [6-oz.] bunch)

1 tablespoon finely chopped garlic

1 tablespoon unsalted butter

3/4 teaspoon kosher salt

Directions

Preheat oven to 400°F. Toss together butternut squash and 1 tablespoon of the oil on a baking sheet; spread in an even layer. Roast until almost tender, about 8 minutes. Set aside.

While squash roasts, stir together hazelnuts, lemon zest, half of the Parmesan, and 1 teaspoon of the thyme in a small bowl; set aside.

Heat remaining 2 tablespoons oil in a large Dutch oven over medium-high. Add mushrooms; cook, undisturbed, until bottoms start to brown, about 5 minutes. Stir, and continue cooking, stirring occasionally, until golden brown and tender, about 8 minutes. Add chard, garlic, and remaining 1 teaspoon thyme; cook, stirring constantly, until chard wilts, about 2 minutes. Add roasted squash; stir to combine. Remove mixture from heat; stir in lemon juice, butter, salt, and remaining cheese until combined. Divide mixture evenly among 4 bowls; sprinkle with hazelnut mixture. Serve immediately.

30.   Sausage & Kale Strata

This take on a classic casserole is hearty but won't weigh your guests down. Gruyère, sausage, and kale is a great seasonal combo; swapping in wholegrain bread adds extra nutrition and staying power. Assembling everything the night before gives the bread the chance to soak up the liquid.

Active: 20 mins

Total: 1 hr 30 mins
 Yield: Serves 12

Ingredients

1 tablespoons olive oil

1 pound mild or hot Italian turkey sausage, casings removed

1 cup chopped yellow onion

2 (4-oz.) bunches Lacinato kale, stemmed and thinly sliced

2 cups 2% reduced-fat milk

1/2 teaspoon dry mustard

1/2 teaspoon kosher salt

1/4 teaspoon black pepper

8 large eggs

1 (16-oz.) hearty whole-grain bread loaf, cut into 1-in. cubes

Cooking spray

4 ounces Gruyère cheese, shredded (about 1 cup), divided

Directions

Heat oil in a large nonstick skillet over medium-high. Add sausage and onion; cook, stirring often, until sausage is browned and onion is tender, 6 to 8 minutes. Stir in kale, and cook until wilted, about 1 minute. Remove from heat, and let cool 5 minutes.

Whisk together milk, mustard, salt, pepper, and eggs in a large bowl.

Combine bread cubes and sausage mixture in a 9x13-inch baking dish coated with cooking spray. Pour milk mixture evenly over bread mixture, pressing gently to submerge bread in liquid. Sprinkle evenly with cheese; cover with lightly greased (with cooking spray) aluminum foil, and chill at least 8 hours or up to overnight.

Remove dish from refrigerator; let stand 30 minutes. Preheat oven to 350°F. Bake in preheated oven, covered, for 30 minutes. Uncover and bake until lightly browned and set, about 15 minutes. Let stand 10 minutes before serving.

Prep this the day before and sleep in a little the next morning!

Conclusion

To conclude, Optavia diet program is result oriented and well-balanced weight loss program, and has gained so much of popularity in the industry over the past 45 years. It is very effective and you will start seeing the results in the first week itself. The diet program has assisted millions of individuals in losing and controlling their weight. The portion controlled meals are convenient to consume, and you can get over the burden of grocery shopping and food preparation. You can reheat the food just before consuming that is all, you do not have to do anything else. Stop thinking. Start taking action and lose weight.

Meal replacements are at the center of this low-calorie diet. This may appeal to some since it largely eliminates the need for most planning, shopping, and food prep. However, individuals who prefer freshly prepared food and variety in their diet are not likely to find the program sustainable or realistic.

The Optavia Diet does address more health concerns, lifestyle conditions, and age groups than most other commercial diet programs, but special populations, particularly those with diabetes, should always consult a physician before making changes to diet.

CPSIA information can be obtained
at www.ICGtesting.com
Printed in the USA
BVHW041038120721
611731BV00016B/696

9 781802 431315